Tanja Mannhart
Tanja Senders
Prof. Dr. Adrian Steiger

Stray animal population management

Tanja Mannhart
Tanja Senders
Prof. Dr. Adrian Steiger

Stray animal population management

A catch-neuter-release project for free-roaming dogs and cats in Rhodes, Greece: Problem analysis and effectiveness of the strategy

Südwestdeutscher Verlag für Hochschulschriften

Impressum / Imprint
Bibliografische Information der Deutschen Nationalbibliothek: Die Deutsche Nationalbibliothek verzeichnet diese Publikation in der Deutschen Nationalbibliografie; detaillierte bibliografische Daten sind im Internet über http://dnb.d-nb.de abrufbar.
Alle in diesem Buch genannten Marken und Produktnamen unterliegen warenzeichen-, marken- oder patentrechtlichem Schutz bzw. sind Warenzeichen oder eingetragene Warenzeichen der jeweiligen Inhaber. Die Wiedergabe von Marken, Produktnamen, Gebrauchsnamen, Handelsnamen, Warenbezeichnungen u.s.w. in diesem Werk berechtigt auch ohne besondere Kennzeichnung nicht zu der Annahme, dass solche Namen im Sinne der Warenzeichen- und Markenschutzgesetzgebung als frei zu betrachten wären und daher von jedermann benutzt werden dürften.

Bibliographic information published by the Deutsche Nationalbibliothek: The Deutsche Nationalbibliothek lists this publication in the Deutsche Nationalbibliografie; detailed bibliographic data are available in the Internet at http://dnb.d-nb.de.
Any brand names and product names mentioned in this book are subject to trademark, brand or patent protection and are trademarks or registered trademarks of their respective holders. The use of brand names, product names, common names, trade names, product descriptions etc. even without a particular marking in this work is in no way to be construed to mean that such names may be regarded as unrestricted in respect of trademark and brand protection legislation and could thus be used by anyone.

Verlag / Publisher:
Südwestdeutscher Verlag für Hochschulschriften
ist ein Imprint der / is a trademark of
OmniScriptum GmbH & Co. KG
Heinrich-Böcking-Str. 6-8, 66121 Saarbrücken, Deutschland / Germany
Email: info@svh-verlag.de

Herstellung: siehe letzte Seite /
Printed at: see last page
ISBN: 978-3-8381-0546-8

Zugl. / Approved by: University of Berne, Vetsuisse Faculty, Division of Animal Housing and Welfare, Doctoral thesis 2007

Copyright © 2009 OmniScriptum GmbH & Co. KG
Alle Rechte vorbehalten. / All rights reserved. Saarbrücken 2009

Table of content

Summary	3
Introduction	5
Animals and methods	6
.... Local demographic, legal and political situation	6
.... Opening of a clinic	7
.... Choice of a catch-neuter-release program	7
.... Method to count cats	7
.... Method to count dogs	8
.... Questionnaires to analyse the roots of the stray problem	8
.... How the survey was carried out	8
.... The catch-neuter-release program (CNR)	9
.... Establishment of the program's effectiveness	9
Results	10
.... Initial cat count	10
.... Initial dog count	11
.... Results of survey questionnaire	11
.... Catch – neuter – release program; results from 42 cat colonies	14
.... Average age division per colony	14
.... Observations of 42 colonies during four quarters between Sept. 2005 and Aug. 2006	14
.... Number of cats found pregnant during surgery, and number of removed fetuses	15
.... Average number of fetuses per pregnant cat	16
Discussion	17
.... Stray dogs	18
.... Stray cats	18
.... Conclusion	21
Acknowledgments	22
References	23
Appendices	25

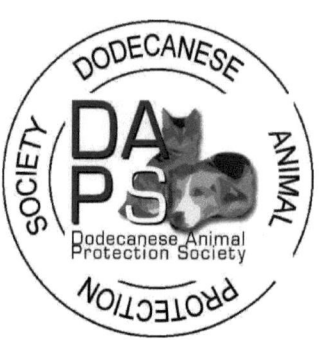

Summary

A new law (law 3170 - FEK/Government Gazette 191/29.07.03), which was proposed by the Greek Ministry of Agriculture, and adopted in 2003 by the Greek government, should obligate municipalities to approach the stray problem according to internationally acknowledged guidelines. Two years after publishing, in Rhodes and the surrounding Islands, the new law had not yet been applied and projects did not show the expected success. Supported by international funds, DAPS (Dodecanese Animal Protection Society), which was represented by a group of young and motivated people coming from The Netherlands, Switzerland and Greece, started a veterinary clinic in cooperation with local authorities in Rhodes, and performed for one year a catch-neuter-release project on ownerless cats and dogs.

The study on "A catch-neuter-release project for free-roaming dogs and cats in Rhodes, Greece: Problem analysis and effectiveness of the strategy" was performed parallel, from September 2005 – August 2006. It analyzes the origin of the stray dog and cat problem in the Greek Islands, and reports about the success of our approach.

Defined areas of the city of Rhodes were initially selected to estimate the number of free roaming cats and dogs in urban areas. In a next step, 75 citizens participated in a questionnaire survey, to gather information about the etiology of the stray problem according to the citizenry. DAPS then worked for one year on a catch-neuter-release project. In total, 1151 free roaming cats and 102 dogs were caught, neutered and released where they were picked up. We collected information on each animal about general health, estimation of age and in case of pregnancy, number of fetuses that were removed. Out of 100 cat colonies, 42 were chosen for further examination on population dynamics.

In urban areas of Rhodes, approximately 778 cats and 29 dogs roam free per square kilometer. Among these, 2.7 % of cats and 24.6 % of dogs are owned animals (pets). 26 % of pet cats and 23 % of pet dogs roam free in the streets and are non-sterilized.

Although over 50 % of the people surveyed valued a neutering campain for strays as necessary, only 44.7 % of pet cats and 37.5 % of pet dogs are neutered, and hardly any are chipped/registered (4.6 %). 69.3 % of the citizens feed street animals regularly. 95 % have observed strays eating from garbage containers and 77 % witnessed poisoning of dogs or cats. Population studies within 42 cat colonies showed, that only 30 % of cats live longer than 3 years, while general health was fairly good. By neutering 84,3 % of the individuals and removing in total 278 fetuses with an average of 4 fetuses per pregnant cat, the population size decreased slightly by end of the one year sterilisation program.

While exhaustive and long-term neutering campaigns are the method of choice in reducing the number of stray cats, the problem of free roaming dogs, which is less severe than the cat problem, needs to be tackled mainly by education programs which create awareness of responsible pet ownership.

The project was disturbed by the continuous hostile attitude of a few local veterinarians, and was therefore abruptly interrupted after only one year.

Introduction

Stray dogs and cats in urban centers and neighbourhoods are a common sight on the Greek Islands. The sexually intact cat population in particular tends to grow out of control, because people with strong affection for these animals feed them. The population size of stray dogs and cats can, however, only grow up to the point of ecological balance. Growth limiting factors are mainly scarcity of food and roaming territories (1). Once a territory is overcrowded, infectious diseases cause increased deaths. Other factors that cause high cat and dog mortality in Greece are street accidents and poisoning. Most local citizens are concerned about animal welfare, yet an excessive number of stray animals can be a source of problems for the public. These animals can transmit zoonotic agents, cause infectious diseases to privately owned cats and dogs, pollute areas with faeces, cause nuisance, for instance through barking, endanger wildlife, and can lead to street accidents where human life may be endangered (1, 2, 5, 6, 7, 8, 12).

Two different methods of stray animal population control exist, which are both recommended by the European Convention for the Protection of Pet Animals of 1988 (3). The catch-removal method takes individual animals from their environment, either by sheltering and rehoming them or by humane euthanasia. The European Convention supports this method only if unavoidable in the framework of national disease control programmes (3). The World Health Organization (WHO) consider this technique alone as ineffective. The catch-removal tactic, without habitat control can have the opposite effect. The population turnover even at highest recorded removal rates is easily compensated for by increased survival rates (4). The second approach is the catch-neuter-release method, by which animals are caught, neutered and afterwards brought back to their natural environment (1-8, 10, 14-16).

According to WSPA (World Society for the Protection of Animals), animal population control must be performed on different levels including legislation, registration/ identification, garbage control, habitat control, neutering of pets and stray dogs and cats, control of breeders/sales, and education of the public (5,6). A new Greek legislation was published in 2003 (Law 3170 - FEK/Government Gazette 191/29.07.03) that legitimizes the catch-neuter-release program to deal with existing problems of stray animals. The responsibility for animal population control projects now rests with Greek municipalities; these projects have to be executed in collaboration with veterinarians and animal protection organisations. With this law, Greece opened up new opportunities to investigate the scope of the stray animal population and ways to deal with this problem keeping the animals' welfare in mind.

Evaluative studies are essential for the selection of a protocol for controlling stray dogs and cats, and may lead to a different approach for each species. The purpose of the study reported here was to evaluate the roots of the stray cat and dog problem and to monitor the success of a catch-neuter-release program on one Greek island. This report should offer a practical guideline to Non Government Organizations (NGO's) and municipalities for a successful population control program.

Animals and Methods

Local demographic, legal and political situation

The project was performed on the Greek Isle of Rhodes, which at 1398 square kilometers is one of the largest of the Greek Islands. Rhodes counts 115'000 inhabitants, of whom 50% live in the capital city, Rhodes, where the study was performed. One of our concerns was to respect Greek laws. To achieve a legal status in Greece, time and money consuming steps had to be taken initially, such as the foundation of a non profit organisation, cooperation agreements with local authorities, the obtaining of licences and the setting up of a veterinary clinic among many others. The project was run under the Dodecanese Animal Protection Society (DAPS).

Opening of a clinic

DAPS received a license to open a veterinary clinic in July 2005. As two veterinarians (Tanja Mannhart and Tanja Senders) we located an appropriate building in Kalithea and furnished it with the help of private funds, financial contributions and donations of surgical materials and medications. This clinic was ready to open in August 2005. A number of large foundations supported the clinic's efforts (see acknowledgment).

The idea to offer practical positions to veterinary students led to a large flow of students from the universities of Utrecht and Bern. At DAPS they had the possibility to gather first hand experience in medical care and surgery under veterinary supervision, while students were willing to help with daily duties. Very soon, the inquiry was higher than open positions. Beside that, some local citizens offered us their help.

Choice of a catch-neuter-release program

Sheltering and rehoming of a projected huge number of animals seemed unrealistic, and massive euthanasia was against our philosophy. In order to be able to establish the potential effectiveness of this program we deemed it important to obtain an estimate of the existing stray dog and cat populations. In light of the seasonal presence of tourists, the cat population typically rises in the tourist season, when volunteers make an effort to feed them. Hence the estimation portion of this project was carried out during the winter months.

Method to count cats

Within the old section of Rhodes town, one area was selected. Twelve overlapping zones with a radius of 150 meters each were drawn. In each zone the observed cat colonies were counted as well as the number of individual cats belonging to each colony *(table 1)*. Selection time for this observation was feeding time, which was determined with the feeders in advance. In order to arrive at reliable numbers, these observations were repeated an average of 6 times. Because the colonies tended to be fed by local citizens at a regular time, the chance to obtain an accurate count were thus optimized. Knowing the caretakers of the colonies was necessary to collect precise data on population dynamics.

Method to count dogs

Within five defined areas of Rhodes (Mandraki, Old town, Kanada street, Hospital-Mengafli, Karakonero-Reni; see *table 2*) stray dogs were photographed and checked with a chip reader for the presence of a microchip. The photocapturing was performed in each area an average of 10 times, until no new dog was seen. The results provided us with an estimate of the average number of dogs per square kilometer (km^2).

Questionnaires to analyse the roots of the stray problem

Questions that focused on the etiology of the stray problem according to the citizenry were developed. With this survey we aimed to obtain information about:
- Attitudes of local petholders, that could influence the stray problem.
- Behavior of local people regarding stray animals.
- Waste management in the city and citizen's awareness of this management.
- The number of pet dogs and cats in Rhodes.
- The way stray animal control had been performed previously.

How the survey was carried out

A sample of 75 local citizens in the street of Rhodes agreed to give answers to our questions. All the interviewing was held during different times of day by the same person in the Greek language. Only one out of 20 people refused to participate, while most citizens were very interested in participating. An effort was made to get a representative sample of different ages of males and females. 31 males and 44 females volunteered for the questionnaire with an age division of 21.3 % < 30 years, 37.3 % 31 – 50 years and 41.3 % > 50 years old. One interview lasted about 10 minutes.

The catch-neuter-release program (CNR)

For one year, the DAPS clinic was occupied with sterilisations and castrations of free roaming cats and dogs. A team left every day to catch animals from the street. Neutering of dogs was not our priority, because a reduction of free roaming dogs needed to be addressed by other measures, as we found out with the questionnaires. In total, 1151 stray cats and 102 dogs were caught and went through surgery (anesthesia with Xylazin 2%, 2mg/kg and Ketamin 10%, 10mg/kg), and then released, after proper recovery, at the same place where they were caught. Each animal was treated for parasites (Ivermectine 0.2mg/kg, Fipronil), received a painkiller (Meloxicam 0.2 mg/kg) and long acting antibiotics (long acting Penicilline, 30 000 U.I./kg), and was registered with a photograph and data about general health, estimation of age (based on teeth observation (9)) and in case of pregnancy, number of fetuses that were removed. Our intention was to get an idea about the life expectancy of the strays in Rhodes.

Establishment of the program's effectiveness

Before surgery every anaesthesized cat was marked with a colony specific number tatooed in the right ear. To avoid recapturing, we cut a tip of the right ear while under anaesthesia. Very sick animals had to be euthanized. Out of 100 cat colonies, we chose 42 for further examination of further data on population dynamics. Between September 2005 and August 2006, clinic staff undertook regular visits to the colonies to determine: a) the total number of cats in the colony, b) the proportion of neutered to non-neutered cats, and c) the number of new arrivals / disappeared cats. The data were categorized into four quarters.

Results

Initial cat count

An average number of 55 cats live in the old town of Rhodes within 1 zone with a radius of 150 m. Within the whole cat counting area, the 12 overlapping zones together, we detected 26 different cat colonies. By overlapping 12 circles of counting, colonies that deviated did not have a large impact on the average number (table 1). Based on these results, we estimated a total number of 778 free cats per square kilometer (km²): (Area = $r^2 \times \pi$ = 70'685.83 m²; 1'000'000: 70'685.83 m² = 14.147; 55 x 14.147 = **788 cats**).

Zone 1-12 of cat counting	Total number of counted cats per zone
1	15
2	93
3	61
4	79
5	77
6	16
7	44
8	60
9	51
10	38
11	99
12	28
Total all zones	661 : 12 = 55

Table 1: Countings of free roaming cats in the Old town of Rhodes, within 12 overlapping zones of a radius = 150 m each.

Initial dog count

Per 1.5 km² we counted a total of 44 stray dogs (*table 2*). These dogs were not chipped, and could not be identified as pets. This translates into approximately **29** stray dogs per km² in Rhodes town.

Area of dog counting	Size of the area in km²	Number of counted dogs
Mandraki	0,35 km²	19
Old town	0,5 km²	8
Kanada street	0,06 km²	7
Hospital-mengafli	0,36 km²	4
Karakonero-reni	0,2 km²	6

Table 2: Results of the counting of free roaming dogs within 5 areas of Rhodes town.

Results of survey questionnaire

From 75 people interviewed, we received the following answers to our survey questions.

With question 1, we wanted to get information about the public opinion, how to solve the stray problem: "What kind of measures should be taken to reduce the stray animal problem?"

	Sterilisation / castration campaign	Sheltering, rehome	Poison	Not necessary to reduce strays	Don't know
Number of answers	39	13	2	8	13

Table 3: Public opinion, how to solve the stray problem.

The majority of people expressed that neutering was the only measure to cope with the stray problem, followed by sheltering and rehoming. Eight people did not see the necessity to handle the stray problem. In particular in the old town of Rhodes, people stated that stray cats were needed to keep the population of mice and rats within limits *(table 3)*.

With question 2, we wanted to know whether they owned a pet (dog or cat), and if yes, how serious they took their responsibilities to chip, neuter and keep their pets restricted. People answered as follows:

Number of pets owned by 75 people	Neutered fraction	Chipped fraction	Fraction wearing a collar	Free roaming fraction	Free roaming + not neutered fraction
38 Cats	17	2	7	17	10*
48 Dogs	18	2	14	15	11**

Table 4: Attitude of petowners, to fulfil obligations, concerning chipping, neutering and keeping the pet restricted. (*) 5 ♀, 5 ♂ (**) 5 ♀, 6 ♂.

All citizens who said that their own pet wasn't taken for sterilisation were asked for the reason why not. The two main answers were that neutering was against the animals' nature, and that the cost of surgery at local vets was too high. Five out of the 75 people mentioned that their veterinarian advised not to have the pet sterilized before an initial littering. According to the questionnaires, 31% of the pet dogs and 45% of the cats were entirely or partially unrestricted, and have the possibility to roam free in the streets. 26% of pet cats and 23% of pet dogs are free roaming and non-sterilized. People also reported that kittens and puppies were frequently dumped in garbage containers. The questionnaire revealed that 52 out of 75 (69.3%) of citizens regularly fed a large number of dogs or cats in the street. This finding is supported by the observation that all stray animals caught and neutered at the clinic were very well fed *(table 5)*.

	Total quantity of free roaming dogs/cats, reported to be fed by 75 persons.	Neutered fraction
Cat	600	150
Dog	46	13

Table 5: 75 persons were asked about the number of free roaming cats and dogs they tend to feed regularly in the streets, and if known, the approximately neutered part.

A comparison of table 4 and 5 reveals that 17 (2.7 %) out of 600 free roaming cats and 15 (24.6%) out of 46 free roaming dogs were owned by someone (pet animals).

In Rhodes, all organic waste is thrown away into the public garbage bins which are located in the streets. Seventyone out of 75 (94.6 %) people questionned reported to have frequently seen stray dogs and cats eating from these garbage bins. Fiftyone people (68 %) said that people let the covers of the garbage open, 31 (41.3 %) noticed that bins were often overfull, so the covers could not be closed and 21 (28 %) stated that the cans lacked covers altogether. Garbage collection was reported to happen daily.

Fiftyeight (77.3%) out of 75 people reported to having been a witness to poisoning of stray animals. Three mentioned that their own pet had been poisoned.

Catch – neuter – release program; results from 42 cat colonies

Average age division per colony

Age estimation within our colonies showed following results: Seventy percent of the cats were 3 years and younger, and only 30% lived longer than 4 years *(figure 1)*.

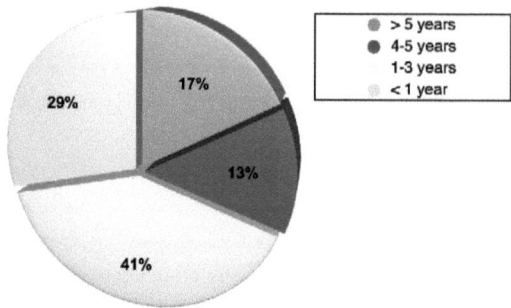

Fig.1: Average age division of a cat colony

Observations of 42 colonies during four quarters between Sept. 2005 and Aug. 2006

Repeated countings during the period Sept. 2005 until Aug. 2006 showed following progress: The number of neutered cats increased from 58 to 575 during this time interval. Close to the end of the fourth quarter, 84 percent of the total cat population was sterilized *(figure 2)*.

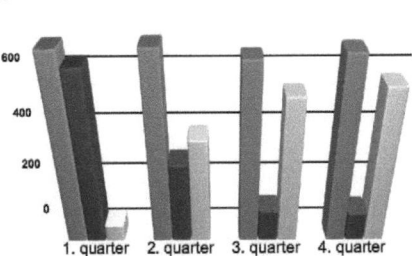

Fig. 2: Results of cat countings, within the 42 cat-colonies. The figure evaluates the changes within 4 quarters of the period Sept. 2005 – Aug. 2006.

Number of cats found pregnant during surgery, and number of removed fetuses

In the 3rd quarter (March-April-May), a very high number of pregnant cats were counted *(figure 3)*. These were neutered before giving birth. A comparison between the cat population size before the neutering program (1st quarter) and towards the end of the program during the 4th quarter revealed a slight decrease from 695 to 682 (1.9 %) cats *(figure 2)*.

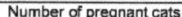
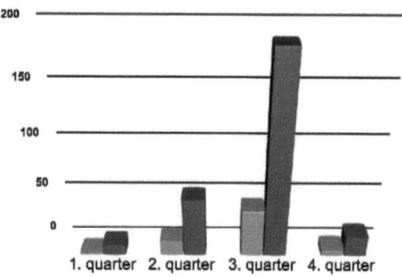

Fig 3: The graphic illustrates the total number of pregnant cats (vertical), which were sterilized during 4 quarters (Sept. 2005 - Aug. 2006), and the amount of removed fetuses.

Average number of fetuses per pregnant cat

While neutering the 42 colonies, a total of 278 fetuses were removed. The average number of fetuses per pregnant cat was 4 (3,97) kittens with a range of 1 – 9 fetuses *(figure 4)*.

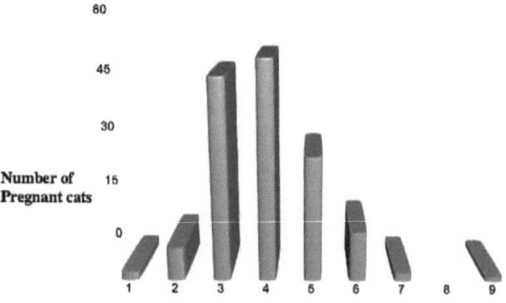

Fig.4: Average number of fetuses per pregnant cat.

Discussion

DAPS received a licence from the Greek authorities to carry out the catch-neuter and release program in 2005/2006. In meetings with governmental veterinarians an understanding was achieved that DAPS would not treat pet animals. Before DAPS started its activities as a stray animal clinic with a spay-neuter program, local citizens of Rhodes used to care for the welfare of free-roaming dogs and cats by offering food or paying local vets for medical treatment, all according to their financial possibilities. Indeed, only a small percentage of strays were lucky enough to get the necessary care, because most people do not have the finances to have stray animals treated or sterilized. With the start of DAPS, free sterilisations and medical care for stray dogs and cats was guaranteed. Out of respect to the businesses of Greek private veterinarians, the agreement to not treat pet animals was strictly honored. Nonetheless, after one year of operation, DAPS had to close the clinic because the ministry of agriculture in Athens denied to renew the annual licence which was necessary to run the veterinary clinic. The same licence we had received one year before, was now suddenly not obtainable anymore. As a consequence we were unable to gather long-term results.

Countings show that Rhodes has a far larger problem to deal with in free-roaming cats (778 / km^2) than in dogs (29 / km^2). We know from the results of our questionnaire survey, that 2.7 % of free-roaming cats and 24.6 % of free-roaming dogs have an owner, even if they are left to roam free in the streets. Many among them are not neutered or micro-chipped and produce regular, unwanted litters. The citizen's enthusiasm of feeding free roaming animals has led to a population explosion of free roaming cats. Other sources of food, such as garbage and tourism, do not seem to be a crucial problem that needs to be approached initially, but should be considered in any long term solution to the stray population problem. The questionnaire points out different priorities to face the stray dog and cat problem.

Stray dogs

Irresponsible pet ownership, meaning neglecting spaying, micro-chipping and keeping a dog restricted, is the origin of the dog problem, and education of pet owners the key measure to be taken. While respecting the business of local veterinarians, spay-neuter-programs do not have access to pet dogs. That is why DAPS did not set priorities on sterilisations of free roaming dogs. Education should focus on the responsibilities of having a pet, and remind owners of the advantages of having an animal neutered. Penalties by government authorities would probably be necessary to motivate responsible pet ownership.

Stray cats

The stray cat population has grown out of control, triggered mainly by the feeding attitude of local citizens. The age divison of cats indicates a very high borning and mortality rate within the cat colonies *(figure 1)*. Target measures for a stray cat reduction are a long term, exhaustive catch-neuter-release program accompanied by creating awareness as to the impact of feeding non-sterilized cats.

Figure 5 describes the population dynamics of a one year sterilisationprogram, within our 42 test cat-colonies. We managed to neuter 84% of the entire population, and removed 278 fetuses, resulting in a slight decrease of individuals by end of the year. Nutter et al. obtained results about populationdynamics in their study on *the reproductive capacity of free-roaming cats and their survival rate* (2). Their findings describe, that a female cat produces an average of 1.4 litters à 3 kittens (4 fetuses) per year, with a 25% survival rate of the first 6 months.

Without sterilisations, in our project around 208.5 (75%) of the 278 fetuses we have removed, would have been born. Considering the 25% surviving rate of the first six months, our colony would have grown by 8.3% by end of the year.

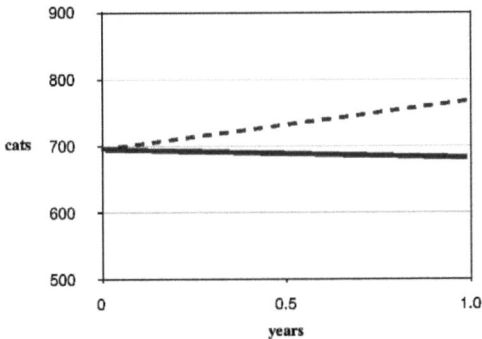

Figure 5: Population dynamics within 42 cat colonies: comparing the development of one year catch-neuter-release program (CNR), and the estimated situation without CNR project.

The lack of long-term results from our catch-neuter-release program has forced us to hypothesize on the development of our 42 cat colonies (figure 6). Assuming that by continuing sterilisations we would manage to avoid future litters, and taking into account our observation that 70 % of our cats die younger than 3 years old, we would expect a population reduction of up to 70% within 3 years. This is also keeping in mind that the life expectation of a neutered colony may rise due to better health and life quality. On the other hand, it is difficult to predict the growth of a non-sterilized cat colony, because their survival is strongly related to environmental factors such as scarcity of food and roaming territories (1). Once a territory is overcrowded, infectious diseases cause increased deaths and keep the population growth in balance. We could therefore expect a seasonal fluctuation in the number of cats, rather than a linear increase, with largest increases during spring caused by litters followed by declines caused by high mortality of the kittens.

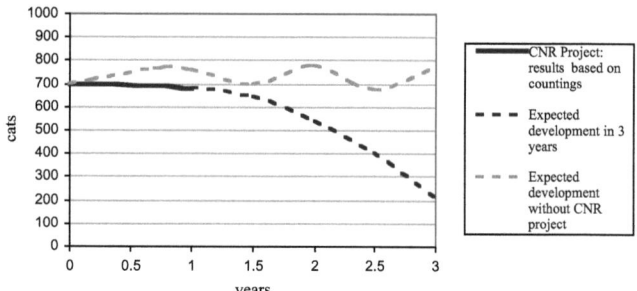

Figure 6: Hypothetic figure of expected long term results. We expect a reduction of up to 70% within 3 years with a long term CNR project. Instable population without CNR project, caused by seasonal littering and high mortality of the litter.

The short term results of a catch-neuter-release program may not be very impressive, but if the program had been continued, long-term results were expected as very satisfying. Once all the females of a colony were sterilized, caretakers could be involved in reporting new arrivals. In this way efforts could be reduced dramatically.

Conclusion

Stray population control programs in Greece are very necessary and welcome by local citizens. Supported by the public, DAPS gained strength and became very popular within the Dodecanese Islands. Citizens from smaller islands sent us their invitations to perform a CNR program on their islands, guarenteeing volunteers and accomodation. The success of DAPS, it seems, caused severe anxiety of several local veterinarians, who used all their connections and power to close the project down. Probably by using such connections, the veterinarians managed to convince the authorities to deny us our licences. The choice to perform a project in Rhodes was very unfortunate because of the presence of these local veterinarians. The same project would probably be successful if performed on smaller islands, where no veterinarians are available.

Acknowledgements

The first author wants to thank all the people and organisations who made it possible for DAPS to exist and work efficiently on the project. Special thanks go to Prof. A. Steiger, Head of Division of Animal Housing and Welfare at the Vetsuisse Faculty in Bern, Toke Hoppenbrouwers, University of Southern California, Los Angeles, Europäischer Tier-Naturschutzbund, Fondation Brigitte Bardot, Swiss Animal Protection, Dutch Animal Protection Society, Greek Animal Rescue, Greek Animal Welfare Fund, Dutch Embassy Athens, Patmos Animal Lovers, Stichting Werelddieren, Animaux, Goutte à Goutte, Een Dier Een Vriend, Boehringer Ingelheim / Vetmedica, Provet AG, Merial, SMI AG, Streuli, Ethicon, AST pharma, Ceva santé animale, Alfasan, ManyMedia, Satz und Druck Lötscher Switzerland, Dierenkliniek De Wetering in Amsterdam and The Waterhoppers dive centre in Rhodes. Further thanks go to all our private supporters, particularly my parents Peter and Magy Mannhart, Lehannah Feric, John Andruchow, the Rhodian authorities Mr. Gonidakis, Mr. Economidis and Mr. Ginis, all our vet assistants and students who joined our project and the Greek citizens who fought with us for the strays of the Dodecanese Islands. Individually I want to express gratitude for the great teamwork with Tasos Manettas, Drs. Tanja Senders and Pier Wouda, Anastasia Kalopetri, Sirpa Newman, Hussein Fetah, Petros Tsoullos and Nina van Wijngaarden.

References

1. Foley P., Foley J.E., Levy J.K.; Analysis of the impact of trap-neuter-return program on populations of feral cats. JAVMA, 227, No.11, December 1, 2005
2. Nutter F.B., Levine J.F., Stoskopf M.K.; Reproductive capacity of free-roaming domestic cats and kittens survival rate JAVMA,Vol 225, No.9, November 1, 2004
3. Council of Europe, European Convention for the Protection of Pet Animals, chapter 3, article 12, Strasbourg 13.11.1987
4. WHO Expert Consultation on Rabies, first report, Geneva, Switzerland, 2004
5. WSPA; Animal control officer: Dog control techniques to assist governmental dept. and municipalities, London, Nov. 1999
6. WSPA; Cat care and control: A practical guide to the management of companion, stray and feral cats, London, 1997
7. Levy J.K., Gale D.W., Gale L.A.; Evaluation of the effect of a long-term trap-neuter-return and adoption program on a free roaming cat population. JAVMA, Vol. 222, No.1. January 1, 2003
8. Andersen M.C., Martin B.J., Roemer G.W.; Use of matrix population models to estimate the efficacy of euthanasia versus trap-neuter-return for management of free-roaming cats. JAVMA, Vol.225, No.12, December 15, 2004
9. Knickel U.R., Wilcek C., Jöst K.; MemoVet Praxisleitfaden Tiermedizin, 4. Auflage, Schattauer Verlag, 2002.
10. Scott K.C., Levy J.K., Crawford P.C.; Characteristics of free-roaming cats evaluated in a trap-neuter-return program. JAVMA,221: 1136-1138, 2002.
11. Centonze L.A., Levy J.K.; Characteristics of free-roaming cats and their caretakers. JAVMA 2002, 220:1627–1633.
12. Feldmann B.M., Carding T.H. ; Free-roaming pets. Health Serv. Rep., Dec. 1979, 88(10): 156 – 962.
13. Lelby L.A., Rhoades J.D., Hewett J.E., Irvin J.A.; A survey of attitudes towards responsible petownership. Public Health Rep. Jul. – Aug. 1979, 94 (4): 380–386.

14 Lerch-Lehmann C.; Bestandesregulierung bei Katzen; in Sambraus H.H. and Steiger A. (Ed.), Das Buch vom Tierschutz. Enke Verlag, 1997.
15 Bögel K.; Bestandesregulierung bei Hunden; in Sambraus H.H. and Steiger A. (Ed.), Das Buch vom Tierschutz. Enke Verlag, 1997.
16 Greek law about stray dog control: Law 3170 - FEK/Government Gazette 191/29.07.03

Appendix

Fotos	26
Questionnaire survey form	28
Satellite picture: area of cat counting	30
Satellite picture: area of dog counting	31
European Convention for the Protection of Pet Animals (extract)	32
WHO Expert Consultation on Rabies, first report; Geneva, Switzerland, 2004	34
Animal protection in Greece, press release about the law 3170	36
Referring articles	38
Educational program proposed by DAPS	42
Final Newsletter	45

Fotos

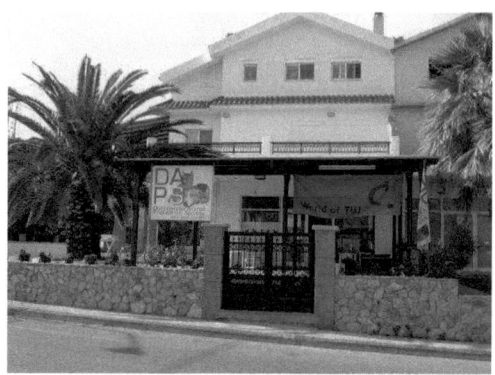

Stray animal clinic of DAPS in Rhodes

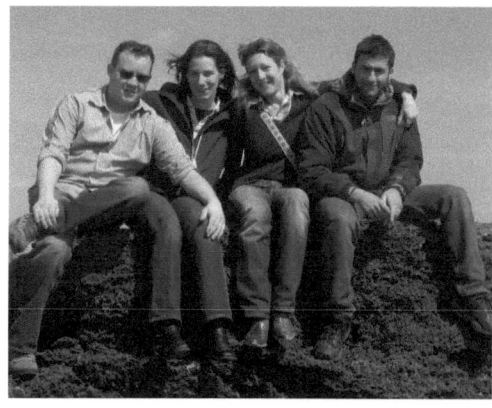

DAPS team (from left to right):
Pier Wouda, Tanja Senders, Tanja Mannhart, Tasos Manettas

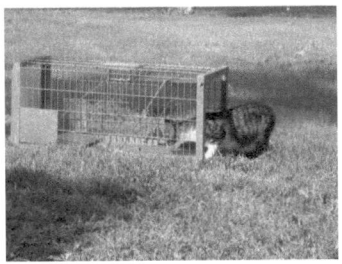 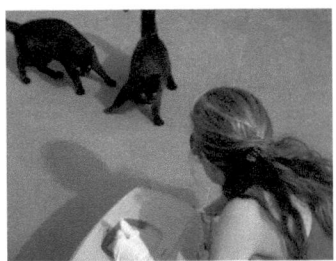

catching cats

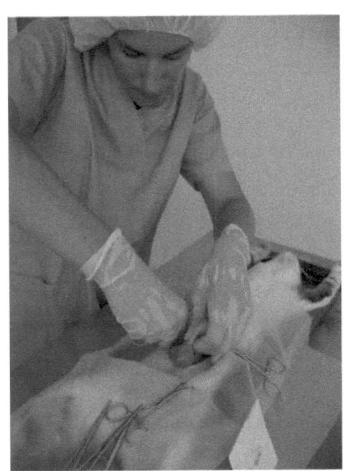 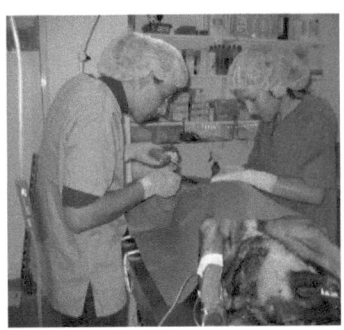

neutering

Questionnaire about stray and pet cats and dogs

Gender: man / woman   Age: _____

Date / Place: _____

_____
[Interviewer make note: describe here loose cats/ dogs in the street, around this address]
_____

[Interviewer make a note of the situation, free standing house, fenced yard (Y/N), apartment like building, how many units, balconies?]

PET ANIMALS:

1. Do you have a dog or a cat in your household?
   a) Yes : dog(s) ____ ♂ ___ ♀ cat(s) ___ ♂ ___ ♀
   b) No : go on with Nr.7

2. Where did your dog/cat stay last night? Yesterday during the day? Where is it now? Is that the usual place that the dog / cat stays during the day and night?

3.a Is / are your pet(s) sterilized , castrated?
   a) Yes: _____
   b) No : _____ why not _____

3.b What do you imagine neutering and sterilization costs in this town/ village?

4. How is your pet marked?
   a) collar __ b) tattoo __ c) microchip __ d) not marked __

5. Did your pet have a litter of kittens/puppies in the past?
   a) Yes: ___ times
   b) Approximately how many were in the litter? _____
   c) No: go on with Nr.7

6. What did you do with the litter?
7. I saw a "shaggy poodle" / white kitten in front of your home, do they belong to someone? (example)

8. Do your neighbours have pets or feed strays?

9. Poisoning of dogs or cats happens a lot in Rhodos. Do you know of an animal that died from poisoning?

STRAY ANIMALS:

1. How do you feel about the stray animals in your neighbourhood?

    a) They don't bother me
    b) I like the idea having animals around that I don't need to take care of!
    c) Negative_____

    → do you have ideas about limiting the growth of the stray animal population?

2. Do you feed any dogs or cats on the street, which don't belong to you?

    a) Yes:
    b) No : go on with WASTE MANAGMENT

3. About how many animals do you feed? Dogs: ____ Cats: ____

WASTE MANAGEMENT:

1. Do you observe stray animals eating from the garbage containers?

    a) Yes: ____ cats____ dogs ____
    b) No : ____

2. Which would you say is the most accurate?

    a) People leave the container open
    b) Containers are often too full
    c) Containers have no cover

3. How often do the municipality empty the containers that belong in your neighbourhood?

    ____ times a week

Counting of cats in the Old town of Rhodes, within 12 overlapping circles (R = 150 m)

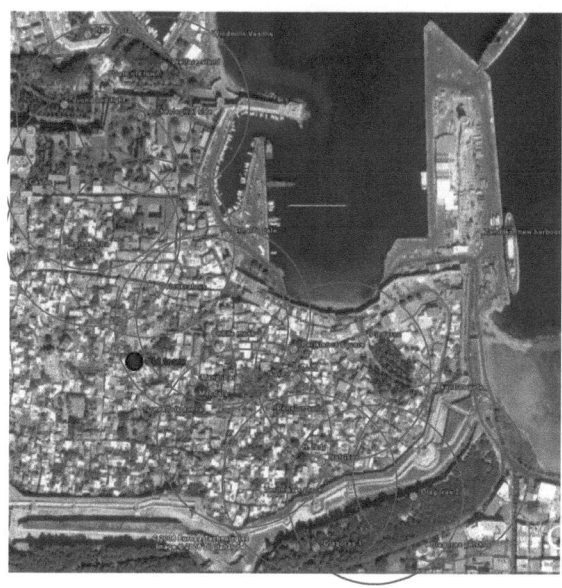

Picture 1: Within the old section of Rhodes town, one area was selected. Twelve overlapping zones with a radius of 150 meters each were drawn. In each zone the observed cat colonies were counted as well as the number of individual cats belonging to each colony.

Counting of free dogs in 5 areas of Rhodes town

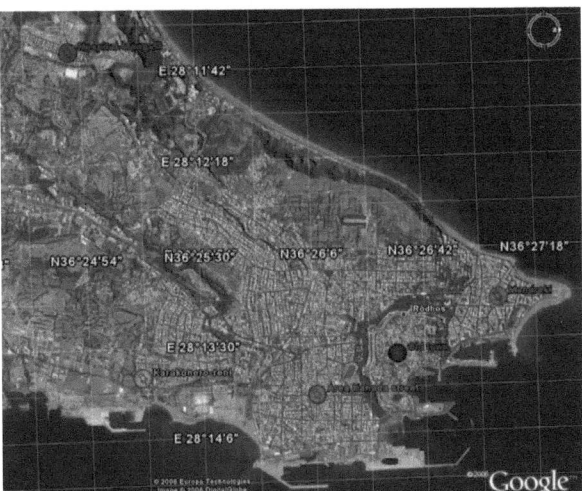

Picture 2: Free roaming dogs were captured by photographs within 5 defined areas of Rhodes city. The photo-capturing was performed in each area many times, until no new dog was seen. With the photos, we could finally count the total number of free roaming dogs in the 5 areas.

European Convention for the Protection of Pet Animals, Council of Europe, Strasbourg 13.11.1987 (extract)

Chapter III – Supplementary measures for stray animals

Article 12 – Reduction of numbers

When a Party considers that the numbers of stray animals present it with a problem, it shall take the appropriate legislative and/or administrative measures necessary to reduce their numbers in a way which does not cause avoidable pain, suffering or distress.

a. Such measures shall include the requirements that:
   i. if such animals are to be captured, this is done with the minimum of physical and mental suffering appropriate to the animal;
   ii. whether captured animals are kept or killed, this is done in accordance with the principles laid down in this Convention;
   iii. Parties undertake to consider:
   iv. providing for dogs and cats to be permanently identified by some appropriate means which causes little or no enduring pain, suffering or distress, such as tattooing as well as recording the numbers in a register together with the names and addresses of their owners;
   v. reducing the unplanned breeding of dogs and cats by promoting the neutering of these animals;
   vi. encouraging the finder of a stray dog or cat to report it to the competent authority.

Article 13 – Exceptions for capture, keeping and killing

Exceptions to the principles laid down in this Convention for the capture, the keeping and the killing of stray animals may be made only if unavoidable in the framework of national disease control programmes.

Chapter IV – Information and education

Article 14 – Information and education programmes

The Parties undertake to encourage the development of information and education programmes so as to promote awareness and knowledge amongst organisations and individuals concerned with the keeping, breeding, training, trading and boarding of pet animals of the provisions and the principles in this Convention. In these programmes, attention shall be drawn in particular to the following subjects:

a. the need for training of pet animals for any commercial or competitive purpose to be carried out by persons with adequate knowledge and ability;

b. the need to discourage:
   i. gifts of pet animals to persons under the age of sixteen without the express consent of their parents or other persons exercising parental responsibilities;
   ii. gifts of pet animals as prizes, awards or bonuses;
   iii. unplanned breeding of pet animals;
   iv. the possible negative consequences for the health and well-being of wild animals if they were to be acquired or introduced as pet animals;
   v. the risks of irresponsible acquisition of pet animals leading to an increase in the number of unwanted and abandoned animals.

WHO Expert Consultation on Rabies, first report; Geneva, Switzerland, 2004

7.4 Dog population management and animal birth control (ABC) programmes

The Consultation expressed its appreciation of the long-term engagement of WHO to contribute to developing methodologies related to dog ecology and dog population management. Considerable experience has been gained in projects coordinated by WHO in Ecuador, Nepal, Sri Lanka and Tunisia and other ecological studies conducted in South America and Asia. However, data collection needs to be continued in other areas and in countries with different social and ecological conditions.

There is no evidence that removal of dogs alone has ever had a significant impact on dog population densities or the spread of rabies. The population turnover of dogs may be so high that even the highest recorded removal rates (about 15% of the dog population) are easily compensated for by increased survival rates. In addition, dog removal may be unacceptable to local communities. However, the targeted and humane removal of unvaccinated, ownerless dogs may be effective when used as a supplementary measure to mass vaccination.

Several methods to estimate dog population densities based on questionnaire surveys and capture/mark/re-observe studies are available (46). The combination of these two methods allows collection of accurate information on the whole dog population and subpopulations, defined in terms of confinement levels or other parameters. Whereas density estimates based on simple capture/mark/re-observe studies using uniform marking (collars and dyes) are usually adequate in rural areas, more complex study designs involving differential or individual marking are recommended in urban and suburban areas in order to compensate for variations in re-observation probability (1). Questionnaire surveys conducted in the community can be useful where residents recognize the dogs present in their communities.

Three practical methods of dog population management are recognized: movement restriction, habitat control and reproduction control.

Attempts to control dog populations through culling, without alteration of habitat and resource availability, have generally been unsuccessful. Since the 1960s, ABC programmes coupled with rabies vaccination have been advocated as a method to control urban street male and female dog populations and ultimately human rabies in Asia. The rationale is to reduce the dog population turnover as well as the number of dogs susceptible to rabies and limit aspects of male dog behaviour (such as dispersal and fighting) that facilitate the spread of rabies. Culling of dogs during these programmes may be counterproductive as sterilized, vaccinated dogs may be destroyed.

Based on 1990 WHO guidelines (*47*), ABC programmes have been launched in several countries and the results have been encouraging, with a reported reduction in the size of the street dog population and the number of human rabies cases. However, data are limited and independent evaluation of projects has not yet been undertaken.

Animal protection in Greece

Press release by the Greek embassy in Stockholm

In accordance with a new bill, proposed by the Greek Ministry of Agriculture and later adopted by the Greek Parliament (Law 3170 - FEK/Government Gazette 191/29.07.03), the responsibility for stray animals in Greece is deputed to the local authorities. The new law establishes:

1. The compulsory tagging and registration of all domestic and stray animals.
2. The collection, sterilization, vaccination and veterinary treatment of stray animals throughout the country.
3. The municipalities and the communities are responsible for the collection of stray animals, assisted by organisations for animal protection. The collection is carried out by specially trained teams, which are under the surveillance of the veterinary authorities of each prefecture.
4. Upon their collection, the stray animals are taken to a shelter, where they, if found healthy, are vaccinated, sterilized and tagged, and where they remain until their adoption. When adoption cannot be arranged, the animals, after a decision of the local authorities, can be returned to their natural setting. They remain there under the surveillance of the municipality, the community and the organizations for animal protection.
5. New laws are being laid down according to which anyone who abandon, ill-treat, torment or exterminate a domestic animal will face a severe penalty.
6. A duty will be paid yearly by the owners of the dogs to the local authorities. The incomes of these duties will be used exclusively for the implementation of a special program for the collection and maintenance of stray animals.
7. New rules regulate the trade in domestic animals.
8. The foundation of new or modernization of already existing shelters for stray animals will be financed by the local authorities or the organizations for animal protection (12 million Euros has been appropriated for the realization of this program).
9. The Greek Ministry of Agriculture and the Organizing Committee of the Olympic Games 2004 have drawn up a program for the dealing with stray animals which rejects the perspective of euthanasia and anticipate the following:

- The collection and tagging of stray animals in the Athens metropolitan area.
- The vaccination and sterilization of stray animals, in cooperation with municipalities and veterinaries.
- The return of the healthy, vaccinated and sterilized animals to their natural settings.

>Also, the Municipality of Athens will allocate approximately 1.8 million euros for the program of protection and adoption of stray animals.

>(Greek embassy in Stockholm, Press release 2004)

Referring articles

Law little help for strays

Authorities are failing to enforce humane population controls for street animals, making a dog's dinner of legislation
CORDELIA MADDEN

NEARLY three years after legislation was passed requiring municipalities to set up sterilisation programmes for stray dogs, only a handful have fulfilled their obligations. Small wonder, then, that the ministry responsible is unwilling, or unable, to provide any
information about the law's implementation. Enacted in July 2003 in an effort to humanely restrict numbers of homeless animals, law 3170 made local authorities responsible for stray dogs, obliging them to set up programmes of vaccination, sterilisation and identification followed by adoption or release onto the streets. On February 20, the *Athens News*
contacted the ministry of rural development, which oversees the implementation of this law, requesting information on how many municipalities in Greece have received funding and set up these catch-neuter-release programmes for stray dogs. To date, despite countless queries to the office of Deputy Minister Alexandros Kontos (under whose authority the issue falls), the ministry has not supplied any data in response to these questions. The only available statistics were gathered by the charity Greek Animal Welfare Fund (GAWF) and the Coalition in Defence of Animals In Greece (CIDAG), members of which conducted a telephone
survey among municipalities last summer. The results make pitiful reading. Of 100 municipalities questioned, only 29 said they conducted stray dog programmes. Of these, 27 ran catch- neuter-release schemes and two operated shelters. With 22 of these municipalities
in the Attica area and four in Thessaloniki, only three others throughout the rest of the country had set up sterilisation programmes. Greece consists of nearly 1,000 municipalities and
communities. Municipalities that conduct stray control programmes include Athens - which says it has sterilised approximately 1,500 and rehomed 270 dogs since the scheme started in October 2003 - Psychico, Agia Paraskevi, Paleo Faliro, Markopoulo, Thessaloniki and Kalamaria, Larissa, and Mytilini. The Lesvos animal welfare group and the former vice-mayor of Mytilini, veterinarian George Paleologos, lobbied the mayor to set up a clinic for sterilising strays. Since December 2004, when it opened, 280 dogs have been sterilised,
treated for injury or illness and identified. "The stray population of Mytilini used to be more than 650 dogs," says Paleologos, "now it's about 150." Half of the 65,000 euros to set up the clinic was paid by the municipality (the other half came from the ministry of Aegean), which also donated the land and pays utility bills. The vet's salary and dogs' medication and food are paid by the welfare society at a cost of

15,000 euros per year. Funding for neutering programmes is a problem. According to GAWF, of all the municipalities that applied for government funding to set up catch-neuter-release programmes in 2004-2005, 17 were informed that their applications had been successful, but only one, Vyronas (eastern Athens), received the funding. Nea Makri municipality, for example, was approved by the ministry for funding in both 2004 (a sum of 11,200 euros for sterilising, vaccinating and identifying 100 dogs) and 2005 (6,000
euros for 50 dogs) but the money never materialised.

No punishments for abuse
Law 3170 cites harsh punishments for those who poison companion animals, but the practice continues unchecked. Since February 2005, the *Athens News* has received reports of mass poisonings on Crete, Corfu, Syros, Skopelos, in Nafplio, Xylokastro, Loutraki, Nea Makri, Porto Rafti, central Athens, Alimos, Dionysos and Maroussi. The latest report was of an
'Easter poisoning' on April 21 of three dogs at a tavern in Thrakomakedones, north of Athens. Yet only one person has ever been found guilty of killing an animal with poisoned bait: in November 2004, George Limakis was penalised for feeding toxin-laced chicken to a neighbour's dog. No one has been convicted for abandoning an animal (illegal since 1981) or for failing to microchip their pet (obligatory since summer 2004). Carol McBeth of GAWF stresses the importance of microchips - and wardens equipped with scanners to check wandering animals - to deter abandonment. Money collected in fines for non-chipping of pets could be used to subsidise sterilisation programmes.
While many welfare societies initially welcomed the law - in most cases they
were already operating catch-neuter- release schemes - they have been disappointed at the lack of results on crucial issues. "The law has resulted in our clinic for sterilising strays," says
Vasso Kazleri of the Mytilini society, "but we were sterilising anyway. If there isn't a welfare group to push the municipality [to implement the law], nothing happens."
Effi Dodoura of Argos concurs: "It's a good law on paper. But it's not enforced."
The groups argue that the current situation hinders their efforts to rehome and sterilise strays, since such responsibilities now fall to local authorities. "The law takes for granted that the municipalities are following programmes for strays, and that all stray dogs throughout Greece have been identified, sterilised and vaccinated," says lawyer Amalia Katsoula. In areas
where there is no municipal programme, she continues, one now cannot "legally" so much as rescue a puppy from a rubbish bin. "The law cannot work as long as there are no municipal programmes: it
must be repealed."
ATHENS NEWS , **28/04/2006**, page: **A09**
Article code: **C13180A091**

New law on collecting and treating stray animals has been allowed to lapse after the Olympics

Plan to have identification microchips implanted in domestic pets and to innoculate, spay and neuter strays has gone by the wayside

The reason there are so many stray dogs around the country - about 300,000, with a third of these in Attica - is that people keep abandoning unwanted litters.

By Lina Giannarou – Kathimerini, Nov. 15 2006

THREE years ago, pet owners rushed to veterinarians for the identity microchips required by a new law (3170/2003) in order to avoid fines of up to 1,500 euros. Thousands of animals were given the microchips and the accompanying documents required for the animals to travel within the European Union. The data bank required to be kept by the Panhellenic Veterinary Society was under way. The prevailing sense was that, in combination with a municipal drive to neuter and vaccinate strays, the plan would reduce the number of stray animals on the streets. The idea was to discourage careless pet owners from abandoning an animal which had the microchip embedded in its skin and which would identify its owner. No one could have imagined that most municipalities would stop collecting strays for treatment immediately after the Olympic Games (when the world's television cameras had gone) and that in the absence of information programs and inspections, owners would not be as conscientious about getting their dogs identity chips. Now their numbers have dwindled to a trickle, while the number of strays on the streets remains high. About 100,000 stray dogs are estimated to be wandering the streets of Attica, with a total 300,000 around the country as a whole. In Athens, there have been fewer strays since the Olympics mainly because of the municipal spaying and neutering program. The City of Athens is one of the very few that have continued with the campaign. However, the reduction in the stray population is not what was expected. According to data from the Panhellenic Veterinary Society, the data bank of microchipped animals currently numbers 90,000 pets; the total number of pet owners, however, is estimated at about 2 million. The main reason for the problem (apart from the lack of awareness about caring for pets) is the complete lack of inspections. In the three years since the law came into effect, the City of Athens Police, which is the authority responsible, has not imposed a single fine. «They have made inspections, but have not caught a pet owner with an unidentified animal,» said the deputy mayor in charge, Tonia Kanellopoulou. «Patrols go out but obviously not when the unidentified dogs are taken out,» she said. Veterinarian Tassos Kanouris scoffed at these claims. «Based on the low number of

animals that have been given microchips, it can't be that hard to find an unidentified animal. I can't understand why they don't carry out inspections, since that would bring in revenue from the fines imposed.» He believes authorities have stopped implementing the pet-related law. «The state has not done what it was supposed to. Apart from taking an animal abroad by air, there are other ways of getting it out without supplying the proper documents. No information is provided. If 60 percent of all pets were brought in for microchips when the law first came into effect, now the figure is one a month,» he said. According to Liana Alexandri, head of the Hellenic Animal Welfare Society, stray dogs are still breeding. «We thought that the new law would help but the problems remain. Animals are still being abandoned. The areas around the Parnitha cable car, Thrakomakedones and the Mesogeia plain are full of strays. Among my own acquaintances who are pet owners, not one has been stopped for a microchip or documents check. If there are no checks, there will be violations of the law,» she said. Greek pet owners are also lax in spaying and neutering their animals. «The main reason there are so many strays in Greece today is the puppies that are still being born both to pets and strays,» said Alexandri. «Owners don't know what to do with them so they just dump them in the streets and [the animals] become tomorrow's strays.»
Kanellopoulou agrees. «People have to realize that they must have their dogs spayed and neutered. It just isn't possible in a European country that people don't realize the need for that,» said Kanellopoulou, who also added that the city would shortly be embarking on a campaign to raise public awareness of the issue. This article appeared in the November issue of ECO, a Kathimerini supplement.

Summary of the Educational programme of DAPS

Goal: Develop the awareness of animal welfare of the children of Rhodes.

Tool: Classes of the primary schools of Rhodes will be invited for an excursion to DAPS.

Overview of the excursion:

Part 1.
Creating awareness of a problem.]
- Showing a movie about the current situation of the strays of Rhodes.
- Starting a short discussion about what the children think about the feelings of animals. Do they feel pain?
- Asking the children if they feel it is important that animals in trouble should be helped, or should we just leave them in their misery?

Part 2.
Explaining the activities of DAPS *during a tour of the premises.*
- DAPS explains its vision on animals, and explains why the DAPS started, and that if no action is taken, the problem will only get worse.
- A tour of the premises of DAPS
- A short trip will be made to a cat-café (a public cat feeding point), where the children can feed the cats, and they can try to find a cat that has not been sterilized or castrated (what can be seen at the tipped right ear). That way the children can actually contribute to the program.

Part 3.
Talking about the responsibility the children have themselves.

- Explaining the very basics of keeping an animal at home.
- Telling the children that they should not think lightly about taking a pet.
- Explaining the pros and cons of keeping a pet.
- Ask the children what they think the benefits are of the DAPS programme. Are only the animals profiting, or are there more benefits?

Maybe the most important thing to teach the children is that animals can be very nice to have around, and they can make life more pleasant and they can bring a smile to your face.

Educational programme of DAPS in further detail.

Main Goal:
Develop the awareness of animal welfare of the children of Rhodes. By doing so the children will understand more about animals in general, and they will know better how to treat an animal, and how to behave when they are around an animal, healthy or sick, aggressive or kind. A side effect is that the wellbeing of animals in Rhodes will improve, and the number of strays on the island will be brought down.

Tools:
Classes of the primary schools of Rhodes will be invited for an excursion to DAPS. The children will have a pleasant morning or afternoon, and they will learn about the wellbeing of animals. Another possibility is that the DAPS visits schools, and motivates school managers or teachers to dedicate a few lessons to the subject of animal protection and welfare. Furthermore flyers will be developed. They will offer general information about animal welfare on Rhodes. The first option, the excursion of the children to DAPS, is preferred. That approach will be focussed on.

The excursion:
Part 1.
Creating awareness of a problem.
- Showing a movie about the current situation of the strays of Rhodes. The children will be confronted with sick animals, animals that are hungry, even in pain. The images that are shown in this movie will be selected carefully, and a committee will judge if they are suitable for children of that age. We want to educate, not to shock.
- Explaining how the problem of the strays started, and starting a short discussion about what the children think about the feelings of animals. Do they feel pain? Can they be sad? Are humans to blame for the problems? Can animals be comforted by humans? Are the children aware of the function of animals? Do they mean anything for humans? (Companionship, guide-dog for the blind, hunting-dog, guard-dog.)
- Asking the children if they feel it is important that animals in trouble should be helped, or should we just leave them in their misery?

Part 2.
Explaining the activities of DAPS during a tour of the premises.
- The DAPS explains its vision on animals, and explains why the DAPS started, and that if no action is taken, the problem will only get worse.
- During a tour through the building the kids are shown what the DAPS does, how the animals are brought in, where neutering/castrating is done, and the children will receive information about why this is useful.
- A short trip will be made to a cat-café, where the children can feed the cats, and they can try to find a cat that has not been sterilized or castrated. (These cats can be recognized by their ears; they have two intact ears.) That cat will be taken back to the DAPS clinic. That way the children can actually contribute to the program. During this trip the children will also be explained to how they should behave

when they find a sick or wounded animal. They can be dangerous, so what do you do? How can an animal that is dangerous be recognized?

Part 3 of the excursion.
Talking about the responsibility the children have themselves.
- Telling the children that they should not think lightly about taking a pet. If they later decide to keep a dog or a cat, they are responsible for the animal for as long as it lives. They are sweet as long as they are young, a puppy or a kitten, but later they can be quite a handful. During this part of the excursion first a puppy or a kitten will be brought in. But later a big grown cat/dog will be brought in, to illustrate that the puppy/kitten will not always be as cute as it is when it's young.
- Explaining the very basics of keeping an animal at home. What do you do? What does it eat? Do you let it in the house? What about the hygiene? How do you behave towards an animal? Can you hit it or kick it? How can you see an animal is healthy and happy?
- Explaining the pros and cons of keeping a pet, like the pet has to be fed, the animal needs a lot of space and exercise, you have to keep it company, and when it has to go to the vet, you have to be prepared to pay for it. And you have registered it through chipping, it has to be vaccinated dewormed and sterilized.
- In the end the children will be asked about what they think the benefits are of the DAPS programme. Are only the animals profiting, or are there more benefits?
- Maybe the most important thing to teach the children is that animals can be very nice to have around, and they can make life more pleasant and they can bring a smile to your face.

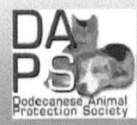

NEWSLETTER
THE FINAL EDITION

DAPS CLOSES THE DOORS

Rhodes, 8th September 2006

Dear DAPS friends, members and sponsors,

As you know, since the 21st of July, the DAPS clinic has been closed, due to problems with the license. So far, we did not succeed in any way to get the license back, and at this point there is no reason for us to believe that we will get it soon. And in spite of all the letters and statements of support that we have received, we took the very difficult but final decision to stop our project. We would like to explain our reasons for that decision.

The most important reason is, as we said, the fact that we have no license to work as vets in Greece right now. The motivation of the authorities to deny us the license, the same license we had last year, is very complicated. And allthough we tried to solve the problem, we had to come to the conclusion that it is too complicated for us both.

Then there is the fact that Tanja Senders announced her withdrawal from the project, in October. This is not unexpected, she initially got into the project for a year, and she stayed for a year and a half. To replace her, we found two young Dutch veterinarians. But to introduce these young vets in the clinic and the project, the clinic needs to be open, and it is not. So we have no chance of properly training the new vets. First we would have to wait for the license, and then Tanja Mannhart would have to do everything alone; the training of the vets, the running of the clinic. And as the person that arranged all our bureaucracy is leaving DAPS as well due too limited time, it all really becomes too much.

Then there is, as allways, the money. Allthough the clinic is closed, and we are not working on animal welfare, we still have to pay the bills of DAPS. And our financial resources are limited. That is another reason to stop now, the money the sponsors gave to us should be used for other projects, projects that are running effectively.

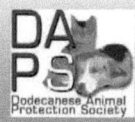

NEWSLETTER
THE FINAL EDITION

And last, but not least, there is the personal motivation. We believe that we had a very successful year at DAPS, from july 2005 until july 2006, we were able to help a lot of animals. But we have spent more than half of our time fighting the bureaucracy, and fighting negative publicity about our work here in Rhodes. And that really made us think. If our hard labour is not appreciated, than we can better bring it somewhere else, it is just not worth it anymore.

We are very sorry about this ending of DAPS, about two months ago we would never have expected this. We hope you all understand that there is no other option for us right now. We thank everybody who has been supporting us the last year, and that have been lots. We hope you will go on supporting other projects that care for the strays.

Sincerely yours

Tanja Mannhart & Tanja Senders

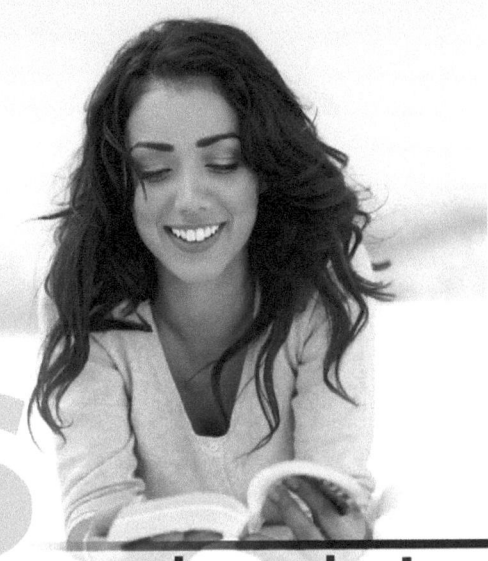

I want morebooks!

Buy your books fast and straightforward online - at one of the world's fastest growing online book stores! Environmentally sound due to Print-on-Demand technologies.

Buy your books online at
www.get-morebooks.com

Kaufen Sie Ihre Bücher schnell und unkompliziert online – auf einer der am schnellsten wachsenden Buchhandelsplattformen weltweit! Dank Print-On-Demand umwelt- und ressourcenschonend produziert.

Bücher schneller online kaufen
www.morebooks.de

OmniScriptum Marketing DEU GmbH
Heinrich-Böcking-Str. 6-8
D - 66121 Saarbrücken
Telefax: +49 681 93 81 567-9

info@omniscriptum.com
www.omniscriptum.com

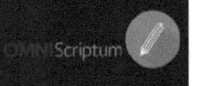

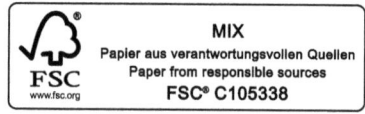

Printed by Books on Demand GmbH, Norderstedt / Germany